Praise for *High Heels to Hormones*

"Christina Lasich, MD, has created a book that is very comprehensive, yet brief and easy to understand. There are many drawings that are humorous, but emphasize important concepts that will be easy to visualize and remember. Overall, this is an excellent self-care guide for anyone with neck or back pain, but is especially written for women."

—James B. Reynolds, MD, Orthopedic Spine Surgery, Chairman and Program Director of SpineCare Medical Group

"Clever and funny ... yet informative, a must read for women of *all* ages. I will incorporate the 'gifts to myself' in my daily life!"

—Cheryl Osborne, RN, MSN, EdD, Professor of Nursing and Gerontology, Director of Gerontology Program and Center, California State University, Sacramento

"Informative and creative ... (*High Heels to Hormones*) is like no other self-help book ... I would highly recommend this book."

—Bob Thompson Jr., PT, DPT, MSPT

"Great gender-specific information for women with back pain ... (this information) is often overlooked or not discussed. (*High Heels to Hormones*) can be a great tool for women."

—Bryan Rodrigues, PT, DPT, MSPT

"Covers a lot of important ground for women with spine pain.... humorous."

—Tim McGonigle, PT

"A fun read with great advice for women."

—John Seivert, MS, PT, GDMT

High Heels
to
Hormones

High Heels
to
Hormones

A Woman's Guide to Spine Care

Christina Lasich, MD

iUniverse, Inc.
New York Lincoln Shanghai

High Heels to Hormones

A Woman's Guide to Spine Care

Copyright © 2008 by Christina Lasich, MD

iUniverse books may be ordered through booksellers or by contacting:

iUniverse
2021 Pine Lake Road, Suite 100
Lincoln, NE 68512
www.iuniverse.com
1-800-Authors (1-800-288-4677)

Because of the dynamic nature of the Internet, any Web addresses or links contained in this book may have changed since publication and may no longer be valid.

ISBN: 978-0-595-46891-1 (pbk)
ISBN: 978-0-595-91180-6 (ebk)

Printed in the United States of America

Cover design by Tracy Tuttle, www.tracytuttledesign.com

This book is intended to be fun, easy, and quick to read for those who do not have the time to invest or the attention span for a more detailed book. For a more comprehensive explanation about this topic, please see the suggested reading list.

This book is not intended to replace professional help but to give you information you might not ordinarily receive in this world of generic medicine for the masses.

For women ready to transform
because pain is a doorway to transformation

Contents

Acknowledgments

It is a pleasure to introduce the contributors to this book. My husband, Paul, is the rock that provides the anchor point in my life. My parents taught me to be brave and independent. My sister is a wonderful mother to the next generation. My friend from grade school, Kaesa, smoothed and clarified my written words. Michelle McKenzie (www.mckenziebookworks.com) provided another set of watchful eyes. Tracy Tuttle (www.tracytuttledesign.com) gave me the confidence to do my own artwork. She also designed the beautiful cover. Bev Phelps took a beautiful picture of me and my baby girl, Pearl. I am grateful to everyone at iUniverse for making this book possible.

Preface

Never underestimate the power of a woman. I saw this on a T-shirt once while visiting the College of William and Mary, except that T-shirt also read: *The College of Mary and William.* Being a young and impressionable woman at the time, I wore that T-shirt until the holes became a bad fashion statement, barely covering the necessary parts. The T-shirt may be gone, but the saying continues to resonate within me. Never underestimate the power of a woman.

Now, as a physician twenty years later, I am conditioned to underestimate the power of being a woman. Very little research is dedicated to studying women's health. However, a gradual onset of awareness for women's health issues has taken place over the past two decades. Breast cancer and cervical cancer have become common household topics as the television blares pharmaceutical companies' wares for treatment. Usually, these commercials air during *Oprah* or *The Today Show.* Men get their prostate cancer and erectile dysfunction commercials during the huge array of sporting events. But cancer and erections are not the only subjects that need gender-specific discussion. Let's talk about the spine.

In the past ten years, I have been a spine care specialist. My practice is filled with women in pain. Sure, I see the occasional male, but the ratio of women to men in spine care practices around the country would make you believe that the male species is rare indeed. If more women have spine pain than men, why isn't there more research dedicated to the study of women with spine pain?

To answer that question, I remember the look on my husband's face when I mentioned that I would write a book about spine care for women. His response was, "Is there a difference?" The response was concerning because, like it or not, many leading spine researchers and caregivers are men. Would they have the same puzzled response as my husband? Are women getting generic treatment for their pain? I hope not, because men and women are different. Those differences have lead researchers to focus on the female spine. Those differences should cause clinicians to address the specific needs of women. Spine care needs to be gender specific.

Being one of those women with chronic low back pain, I know all too well how my female gender influences my pain. I have struggled and sacrificed in order to bring the discomfort under control. The concepts that I would like to present here are derived not only from evidence-based medicine but also from my experiences as a woman with spine pain and as a physician who treats it. Never underestimate what the power of being a woman does to your spine.

Navigation Page

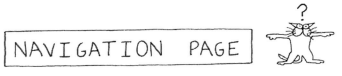

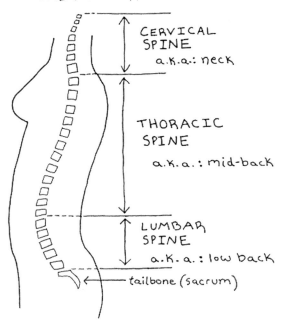

THE SPINE (part of the skeleton)

CERVICAL
SPINE

a.k.a.: neck

THORACIC
SPINE

a.k.a.: mid-back

LUMBAR
SPINE

a.k.a.: low back

tailbone (sacrum)

General Health
For Your Spine

INTRODUCTION

"We can do it!"

This slogan, along with a picture of "Rosie the Riveter," was the battle cry for women during World War II.

I knew a real life "Rosie." Her name really was Rose, and she told me stories about working in the factories during the war. As part of the war machine, she learned how to work with metal.

Years later, we met when I was a firefighter. As the fire station's cook, she could make those pots shine at the fire station where she cooked, cleaned, shopped, and organized her way into our hearts as "CasaRose." No matter how late we got back from a fire or how many mouths she had to feed, she always had a warm, satisfying meal ready for us. Rose's generation was the first to take those multitasking skills from the house to the workforce when women answered the call with "We can do it!"

Often times, this multitasking, "do it all" attitude leads to spine pain in women. Good health is your best defense.

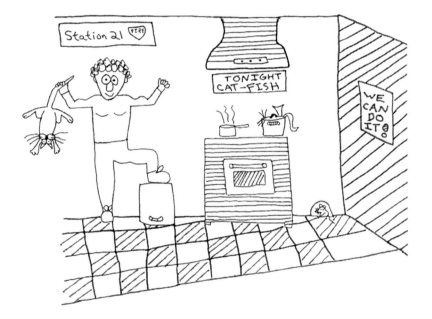

TITLE IX

Historical Perspective

The "we can do it" spirit did not hit athletics until Title IX was passed in 1972.

This federal law states: "No person in the United States shall, on the basis of sex, be excluded from participation in, be denied the benefits of, or be subjected to discrimination under any educational program or activity receiving Federal financial assistance."

Until then, women were discouraged from participating in sports for fear that girls would be physically harmed. Those deterring voices did not know that physical activity for young girls is an important part of developing good body mechanics and good exercise habits.

Prior to Title IX, the only sport a girl could find was through the Girls' Athletic Association, which was mostly disorganized intramural pick-up games. Some girls joined boys' teams just for the opportunity to train, but they were not given the opportunity to receive athletic scholarships. Those opportunities came slowly when Title IX passed.

The spirit of Title IX allows women to "go for it!"

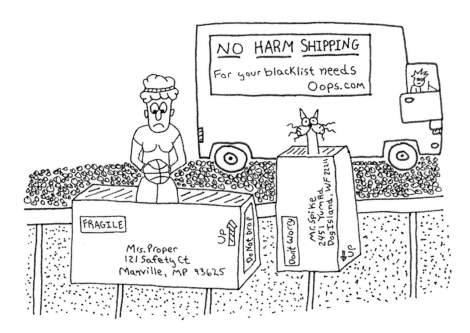

Impact on Spine Pain

Unfortunately, Title IX passed too late to help the baby boom generation. This generation of women did not learn a body language through physical education.

Body language is essentially a roadmap for movement, also called a pattern of movement. Without the necessary patterns of movement laid down during childhood, many women in this generation do not know how to lift, bend, twist, and reach properly. Some are extremely clumsy.

These pre–Title IX women are especially susceptible to spine pain because they entered the workforce without any type of physical conditioning. When spine pain does develop, the women who did not have a positive childhood experience with exercise have difficulty obtaining the proper body language for escaping pain. These women also have difficulty maintaining physical condition through good exercise habits. Good habits are critical for your health.

Just imagine learning a new language. All languages, including body language, are much easier to obtain when you are young. We should be encouraging our daughters to "go for it!"

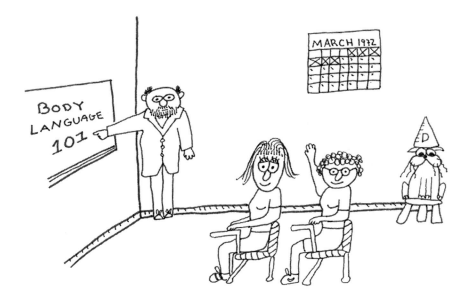

SUFFERING AND PAIN

Reality Check for the Multitasker

"Do it all" is the motto of women who are constantly on the go as the ultimate multitaskers.

When pain and disability set in, a new reality is created by your body's ever-changing ability to tolerate activities—called tissue tolerance. Tissues can only tolerate so much pushing, pulling, squishing, and pounding.

As a survival strategy, your body was born with a high degree of tissue tolerance. Naturally, children have a seemingly unlimited ability to bounce back. Just watch your children in gymnastics. Ouch! It hurts to even think about bending that way! Eventually, aging diminishes the resilient nature of the ligaments, bones, and muscles.

So as you grow older, do not expect your body to have unlimited capabilities. It is equally important to manage other people's expectations of you. The sheer number of requests can become physically demanding. If you keep giving in to others' expectations, the spine will just start pushing back with pain because the spine cannot "do it all."

Just like a checkbook, your spine can only handle so many withdrawals without a deposit. Give yourself permission to "just say no," and you can avoid suffering with pain.

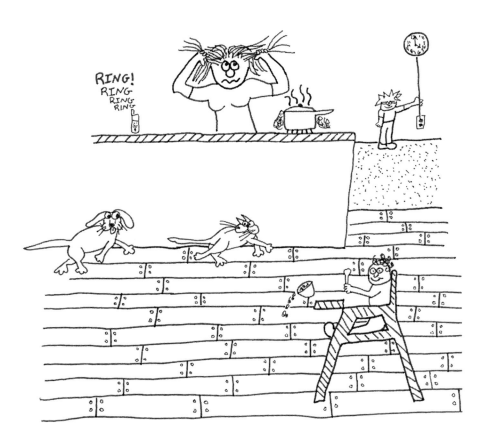

Women as Caretakers

From multitasking to nurturing, how can the ultimate caretakers avoid suffering?

We women are more likely to suffer with pain because of our tendency to be fearful and to worry. We constantly use the past as a source of comparison as we worry about the future.

Have you heard this inner voice before? This fearful voice amplifies any physical pain that may be present such as back pain, neck pain, and headaches. Once the pain is worse, it is then viewed as a threat to the way things used to be and a threat to your continued happy way of life. As a threat, the pain is no longer an annoyance that you can ignore.

Thus we have a cycle: Fear amplifies pain and pain amplifies fear. Pain and fear can run vicious circles around you.

Fear not. Look to your dog (woman's best friend) for advice. And just like your dog, you need to let go of the past, stop fearing the future, and live in the moment. In the moment, you give up desire to remain as you were. In the moment, you do not worry about the future. In the moment, you are released from fear and pain. In *that* moment, the pain will be less threatening.

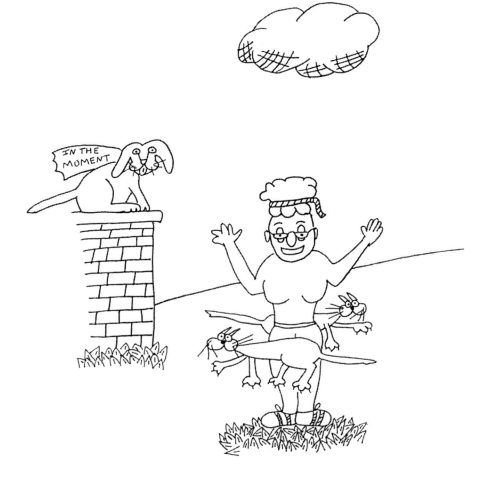

HEALTHY FEAR

Smoking

"No fear" is a popular saying for the young and the young at heart. But having no fear is not necessarily a good thing, especially when it comes to making good, healthy choices. If you decide to smoke, now fear this: Smoking will cause back pain. The more you smoke, the more intense the pain will be and the longer it will last (if it ever goes away). This fact especially holds true for women.

Scientists used to think that the link between smoking and back pain was due to the coughing caused by smoking. However, with the newest research technology, doctors have proven that spinal discs literally dissolve from malnutrition caused by the reduction of blood supply in smokers. The discs also dissolve from the exposure to nicotine.

Wake up and smell the ashes; smoking causes pain. No ifs, ands, or butts about it. It's time to use pain as your motivator to quit this addiction. It's time to educate the young that pain is caused by smoking. Women live with enough pain. Why would you want to smoke your way into constant pain? Instead, try a healthy fear of smoking, and you will save yourself from pain.

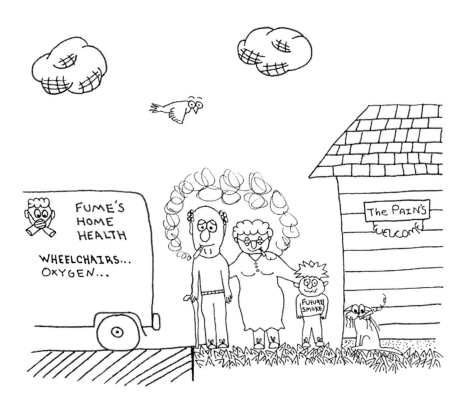

Convenience Food

As a nation, we are addicted to convenience food, but we also need a healthy fear of it.

Women are usually in charge of gathering the food for the household, but who has time? You owe it to yourself and your loved ones to pay attention to the popular saying, "You are what you eat." Let's face it. The chips, sodas, and sweets in the grocery cart eventually end up on the hips, thighs, or bellies.

Grocery carts don't lie about your physique. MRIs don't lie either. Fat blobs take up space in critical back muscles. Fatty muscles are poor stabilizers of the spine and increase your risk of back pain.

Furthermore, a new medical syndrome called "metabolic syndrome" is now linked to high levels of inflammation. If you are obese, have high cholesterol, high blood pressure, and diabetes, you have metabolic syndrome. A combination of metabolic syndrome and high inflammation increases the risk of heart attack and Alzheimer's disease.

Some scientists claim that arthritis and uncontrolled inflammation are caused by diet. Andrew Weil, MD, has gone as far as formulating what he calls an "anti-inflammatory diet" in his book *Healthy Aging*. Convenience foods are not part of a healthy diet. Snack foods may be convenient and comfortable, but these foods are high in sugars, salts, and processed fats (like vegetable shortening). Dr. Weil especially emphasizes the need to avoid sugars and processed fats because both promote inflammation. For a healthy diet, your cart should have a rainbow of colorful fruits and vegetables.

In reality, losing weight with a good diet will provide more comfort than a box of Oreos. Getting away from scary convenience foods just might make us all feel better.

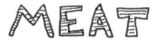

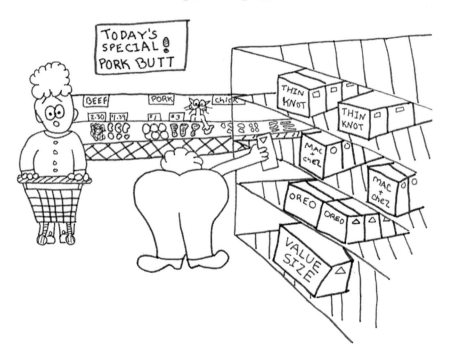

Warrior Syndrome

Two types of exercise warriors exist. One type has no regular exercise maintenance program and uses the weekend to make up for the shortfall. Other warriors do extreme exercise every day.

Either way, the battle can have its casualties: ankles, knees, hips, backs, etc. Each is a victim of too much of a good thing. An injury to one part, say a knee, can lead to future problems below, in the ankle, or above, in the back. Protect these valuable parts with age and condition-appropriate exercise. (You don't win if you die with the most replaced parts.) Being a woman doesn't exempt you from warrior syndrome.

Any form of exercise can be done to extreme. For example, yoga is popular and assumed to be very healthy, but done to the extreme even yoga can lead to disc degeneration and spine pain. Have you seen some of those poses? Ouch!

Women can be smarter than the "no pain, no gain" concept by staying away from extremes and gaining a healthy fear of the warrior syndrome. Tame the woman warrior with a new battle cry, "Gain without pain."

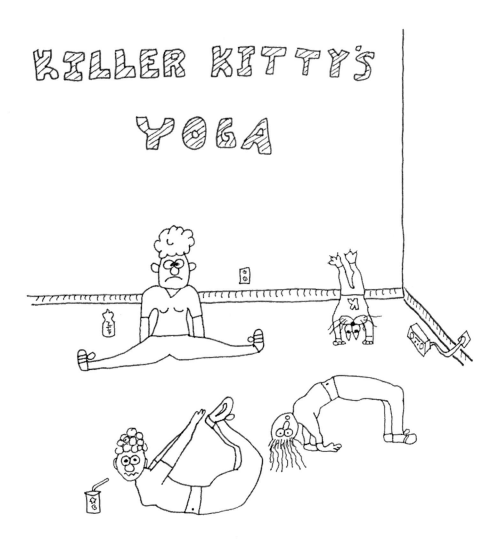

CONCLUSION WITH TWO FOR YOU

Rose's generation is just about gone, but today's women continue to answer with a "we can do it" and "do it all" attitude. Soon the body pays a price, especially the body that does not have a good roadmap for movement.

Take a moment to listen to your battered body. Spine pain does not necessarily have a message of fear or worry. The pain has a message of motivation to become a healthier, better woman. Empower yourself to choose the healthier path by saying no to demands, addictions, and extremes.

Here are two exercises for you to start your journey. Give yourself a gift.

One

Many women suffer from the anxiety and worry of being a caretaker and a multitasker. Try to substitute those negative feelings by finding a mantra to repeat to yourself when the fear overwhelms you.

I have had the same mantra for thirty years, and the final lines bring me back to center: *for thy sweet love remembered such wealth brings; that then I scorn to change my state with kings.*

William Shakespeare works for me; find something that works for you. Your mantra will keep you centered and true to yourself.

Two

Some of you may not have a good body language. Here is a pattern of movement to practice because repetition creates good habits.

HERE KITTY

SQUAT

REACH

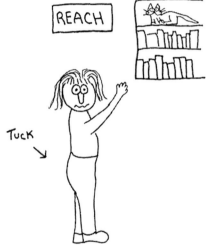

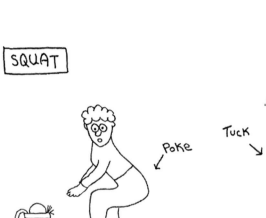

Poke

Tuck

ONE

Reach Below Waist:

① Feet shoulder Width apart
② POKE butt out, Reach
③ Repeat

TWO

Reach above Waist:

① Feet apart
② Tuck tailbone under you, Reach
③ Repeat

Cervical Spine Pain

INTRODUCTION

When your neck hurts, sometimes it feels as if the weight of the world is on your shoulders. Well, that weight is really just your head balancing on top of your painful cervical spine (see the Navigation Page).

Anne certainly felt that way when she came to see me with neck and shoulder pain accompanied by numbness, pain, and tingling into her arms. Even though she did not have a whiplash injury, her pain kept her from fully participating in work at home and at the office. Every time she went bowling, the pain just intensified.

Since her activities became limited, she gained weight. Guess what? Her breasts got bigger and her bra started to make indentations in her shoulders. The pain continued to intensify to the point that her neck could no longer withstand the weight of her own head. Her head was the bowling ball, and she was the bobble-head doll.

Many women, like Anne, have the weight of the world on their shoulders, and they need some gender-specific advice for treating cervical spine pain.

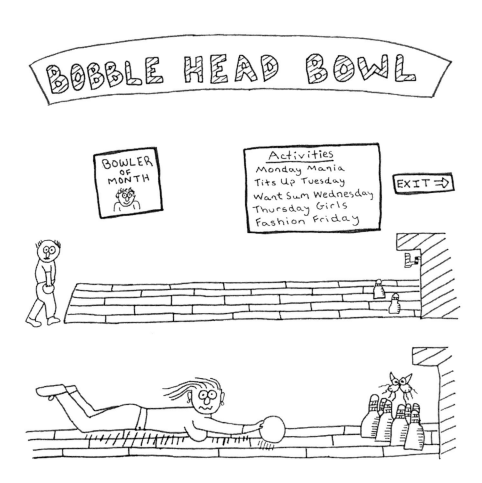

WHIPLASH

Gender Differences

Why do so many women have neck pain?

One reason is that women are more susceptible to whiplash injuries. Our vulnerability is not because we are weak and emotional; our vulnerability is actually due to basic structural differences.

The primary structures injured during a snapping of the neck are the small joints, called the cervical facet joints. These joints are held together by ligaments and protected by cartilage sandwiched between the bones. The facet joints of women move more during whiplash than do those of men, possibly because our ligaments are naturally looser (see Baby Machine section).

As the neck whips around, the ligaments are stretched, and the bones of the joints crush together. Normally, the cartilage offers some protection. Because women were shortchanged in the cartilage department, we actually have less protection for the cervical facet joints than men.

Sorry, gals, you cannot get a refund, but you can get a serious pain in the neck from the stretch and crush of a whiplash injury.

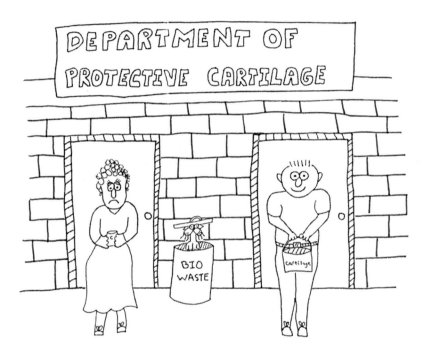

Vehicle Selection and Set-up

Let's talk about prevention, because who wants a pain in the neck? This is where insurance companies should get motivated to help you because they would like to avoid paying for your injury.

Recently the Insurance Institute for Highway Safety (IIHS) issued a report about vehicles and their ability (or lack thereof) to prevent neck injuries. The Volvos and Saabs received the best rating for whiplash protection. But the American vehicles did not fare too well.

I am not saying rush out and buy a Volvo. Just think about being a smart consumer and certainly be smarter than a pain in the neck. Before you buy, check out the IIHS Web site. If you choose a lesser-rated car, at least you should adjust your seat properly. Take the time to check your headrest. The headrest should extend as high as the center of your head. Your head should be in very close proximity to the headrest. This positioning enables the headrest to immediately restrain your head and neck when Junior rear-ends your car.

Like it or not, gender differences do exist in the cervical spine, and women need to give some special consideration and attention to prevention when it comes to whiplash injury.

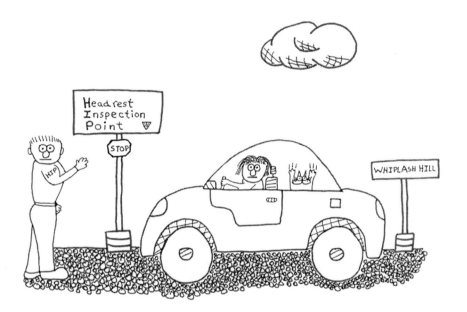

CHEST OUT, LADIES

Base of Support

Besides whiplash injuries, typical neck pain is generated from the base of the neck where the shoulders connect. As the base of support, the shoulders play an important role for the neck.

Because our arms constantly do tasks in front of our chest, the shoulders tend to round forward, and the head follows. As the head comes forward, the weight from the head increasingly stresses the lower neck. Visualize a turtle sticking his neck out from under the shell. Try it on yourself. Notice how the neck arches while the head stretches forward.

I do not know what turtle shoulders look like, but I do know that your shoulders need to stay back with the chest out. Shoulders back, chest out is not just for the military. Find a mirror and strike the "military" pose. Now, notice what happens to the neck. As the shoulders come back, the chin tucks closer to the chest while the neck relaxes into a neutral position. No more turtle!

The ability to find a comfortable, neutral spine position is extremely important for easing spine pain. Because your ability to find the right posture is greatly impaired when the body is injured, injury is more likely to be ongoing until you can accurately find the comfortable, neutral position.

Your accuracy in finding a correct position or pose is greatly enhanced by using a mirror. Thus, all women need a good mirror not just for primping, but also for striking a good pose. When you are done primping, do a body check and make sure your neck is properly supported. Strike the military pose!

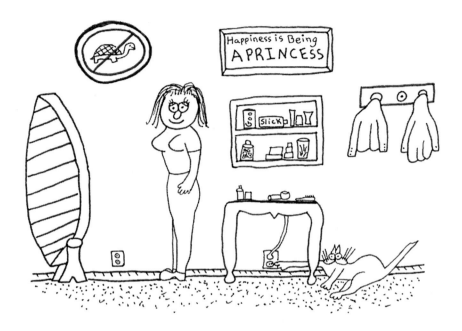

Shyness

No one ever accused Madonna of being shy. Some may remember her costume-enhanced points that threatened to poke an eye out.

Do you remember when you first noticed your breasts forming? Not wanting anyone to notice, some young ladies round their shoulders forward so that the shirt does not cling too tightly. Some women are constantly self-conscious about their breasts.

Unfortunately, breasts are symbolic for sexuality and, in turn, morality. Many people thought Madonna was immoral for the way she flaunted her "girls."

Did I threaten your sense of decency by telling you to stick your chest out with the shoulders back? Pop go the girls, right out for all to notice. Don't be shy, because shyness creates an unhealthy, slouched posture.

Remember, the forward shoulder posture forces the head forward thereby increasing the weight supported by the base of the neck. Ouch!

So keep your shoulders back and be proud of your femininity. This pose is not a morality issue; this pose is a health issue with the intention of saving your neck.

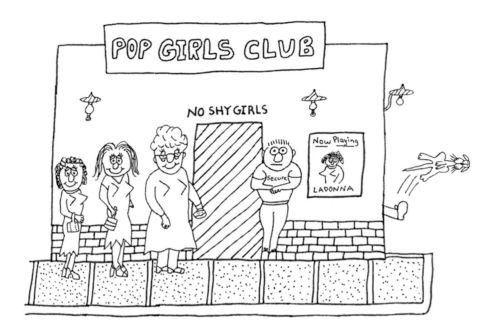

BREASTS

Bras

Speaking of health, some women are confused about whether or not wearing a brassiere is necessary for breast health.

Did you know that bras also influence neck pain? The invention of the brassiere arose from corsets. Corsets were thought to be medically necessary because of the fragility of women. Eventually the corset became a fashion statement and a symbol of a woman's morality. A loose corset symbolized a "loose" woman.

In 1914, Ms. Mary Phelps Jacobs invented the brassiere. Later, Warner Brothers Corset Company bought the bra design.

To this day, bras are a staple item in most women's wardrobes, but at what cost? Some argue that wearing bras can lead to less healthy breast tissue and possibly breast cancer. The link between bras and breast cancer is controversial, but the link between bras and neck pain is clearly established.

In a study by the North American Spine Society and Maidenform, 59 percent of the women who wear a bra say it causes back, shoulder, or neck pain. Clearly, bras can cause indentations in the shoulders. This process is called shoulder grooving. I commonly observe bra straps pulling women into unnatural postures because the straps are supporting pounds of weight. Not only do the straps pull women into the forward shoulder/head (turtle) posture, but the straps also pull the shoulders down, which tugs on the cervical nerves (see Tugging and Shrugging section).

If your breast weight is supported with the bra straps, you need to get a better fitting bra. A good bra should support the weight of the breasts from below with a support shelf. For those with smaller breasts, a fit specialist in a good lingerie department can help you find a properly fitting bra. In fact, Oprah Winfrey's website (www.oprah.com) has great tips from a brassiere specialist. If you have challenging breasts, invest in a custom bra (I recommend Maria Monti with www.thehealthybracompany.com). All women should know that the wrong brassiere can lead to neck pain, shoulder pain, or thoracic outlet syndrome (See Thoracic Outlet Syndrome section).

If you cannot avoid shoulder grooving, burn those bad bras and set your girls free.

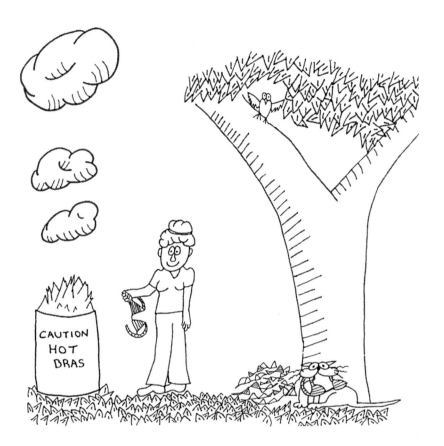

Size Matters

Maybe some of you have large breasts (natural or not) and have difficulty finding the right size bra beyond double D.

You might want to consider downsizing. In fact, the primary motivator for breast reduction surgery is neck and shoulder pain. Large breasts are known to contribute to headaches, shoulder pain, back pain, and shoulder grooving. Not so groovy for those blessed with watermelon-sized girls. The blessing eventually becomes a curse. Some women, artificially blessed with implants, find out later that the pain is not worth their lusty lovelies. (Think before you implant because vanity has a price.)

Those seeking relief from nature's gift will find that this topic is hotly contested. Insurance companies claim that breast reduction surgery is a cosmetic procedure and thus should not be covered by insurance. A court ruling in 1996 created case law that forces insurance companies to pay for breast reduction surgery as a medically necessary procedure offering vast improvements to women in pain. This surgery removes the weight from the front of the chest.

Women have told me that the difference feels like carrying two five-pound sacks of sugar before the surgery versus two apples after the surgery.

Whew! What a difference for the posture.

Whew! What a relief for the neck and shoulders.

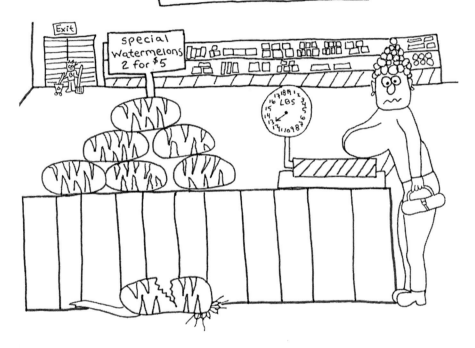

CONCLUSION WITH TWO FOR YOU

Even if you do not have the weight of the world bobbling on your shoulders, you now realize how vulnerable women are to cervical pain. Special precautions can be taken to prevent whiplash injury, a gender-biased problem.

The gender factor does not stop there, however; women especially need to be concerned about how vanity and shyness affect a healthy posture. Cosmetic surgeons and nature bring us large, heavy breasts that weigh the neck down, while shyness brings us caved-in chests as we try to hide these sexual objects.

Freedom from neck pain can come from burning poorly fitting bras, as well as from taking the liberty of sticking your chest out and being proud of your gender. We are a gender that does not need artificial protection in the form of bras or artificial delights in the form of implants. These man-made items create a pain in the neck for women.

Now take a moment to give yourself one of these two gifts.

One

When a mirror is not enough to guide you in finding a comfortable, neutral position for your neck, this exercise can enhance your posture by turning *on* the neck-flexing muscles and relaxing the tight muscles behind your neck.

Two

Some muscles need to be stretched, such as the pectoralis muscles behind our breasts. When these chest muscles shorten, the shoulders pull forward into the dreaded turtle posture.

Try this exercise throughout the day in order to balance out the repetitive forward shoulder position.

TWO

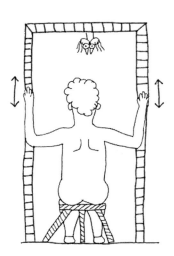

ONE

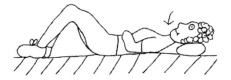

Chin Tuck:

1) Lay On Flat Surface with Head Resting on Pillow
2) Do Not Lift Head Off Pillow
3) Tuck Chin Towards Chest
4) Hold 10 seconds + Repeat

Keep Shoulders Back:

1) Sit in Open Doorway
2) Squeeze Shoulder Blades Together
3) Move Hands up + Down on Door Frame Keeping Shoulder Blades Together
4) Repeat

Thoracic Spine Pain

INTRODUCTION

Sharon came to me with a distraught look on her face. "Please help me! I am starting to look like my mother. I have a humpback."

Sharon's mom had multiple spine fractures due to osteoporosis, and Sharon was worried about developing the dreaded hump as the thoracic spine (see the Navigation Page) curves like a C toward the ground. Osteoporosis is the loss of bone density that weakens bones and causes them to break (fracture).

I had been treating Sharon for thoracic outlet syndrome, which was causing pain, numbness, and tingling into both arms, but her current concern shifted my attention to osteoporosis and prevention of "fragile" fractures caused by the weakening bone structure. After a bone density scan, I was able to direct her and her physical therapist toward some key steps in preventing the dreaded hump. Her improved posture also helped her symptoms of thoracic outlet syndrome. Now, she can wake up, look in the mirror, and not see her mother's likeness.

It is time for you to learn some key points about the mysterious thoracic spine. This part of the spine gets overlooked like a middle child who lacks attention by unwitting parents. The thoracic spine lies between the notorious neck and infamous low back.

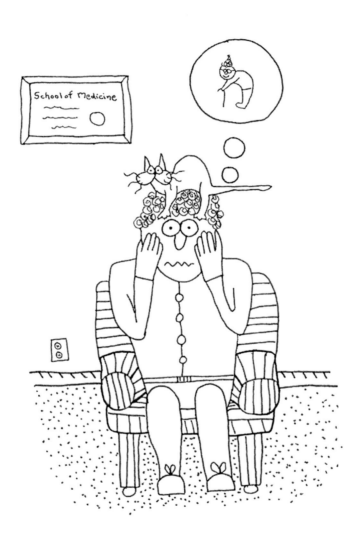

SLOUCHING AND STIFFNESS

Kyphosis

"Don't slouch!" my mother used to say as I headed out the door to school.

Her advice is important because slouching creates a C out of our normally S-shaped spine. In medical terms, slouching is called thoracic kyphosis. The apex of that C is the kyphotic thoracic spine pulling both the cervical and lumbar spine into unhealthy positions. Slouching is viewed as a lazy sitting posture. As the back muscles fatigue, the chest is pulled by gravity toward the knees. The only things stopping you from hitting the floor are your bones and ligaments. And there lies the problem: Bones can fracture and ligaments painfully stretch from the sustained stress of sitting with a lazy, slouched posture.

If you habitually slouch, the abdominal muscles eventually shorten to the extent that you will not be able to straighten up. Over the years, a permanent hump will form in the thoracic spine. Doctors call this the "dowager's hump" commonly seen in women with osteoporosis. As the distance between the bottom of the rib cage and pelvis shortens, the lungs get crowded causing shortness of breath, the stomach gets crowded causing indigestion, and the bladder gets crowded causing incontinence.

So the next time you are sitting at your desk, consider putting up a sign to remind yourself of some good motherly advice and "don't slouch!"

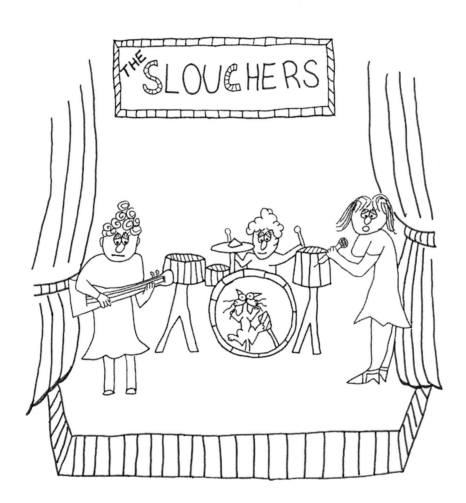

Hypomobility

Hypomobility is just a fancy word for stiffness. Not only is thoracic hypomobility being recognized as a major cause of thoracic spine pain, it is also a contributor to neck, shoulder, arm, and low back pain.

The thoracic spine is truly the common link for many painful conditions of spinal origin. How does stiffness develop?

Sustained postures that limit motion over long periods of time create stiffness. The rib cage itself adds structural stiffness to the thoracic spine. Women seem to be more likely to develop stiffness because of the repetitive nature of our jobs at home and at the office.

When the thoracic spine is stiff as a board, the movement has to come from somewhere else. In order to compensate, the lumbar spine or the cervical spine are forced to move too much. This is called compensatory movement. Compensatory movement causes pain in the neck and lumbar spine because of overuse.

In order to ease these pains, thoracic stiffness must be loosened, and thoracic mobility must be restored. The low-tech way to adjust your own thoracic spine is with two tennis balls in a sock, rolled up and down your spine as you stand with your back against the wall. Self-treatment of the thoracic spine is as simple as that—no frequent trips to the doctor, chiropractor, or therapist. If you are stiff as a board, improved mobility may give you freedom from thoracic spine pain.

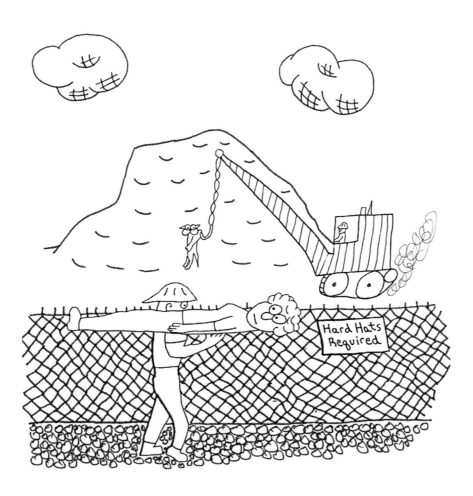

THORACIC OUTLET SYNDROME

Armrests

Women are three times more likely than men to have thoracic outlet syndrome, which is a mechanical irritation of nerves and/or blood vessels under the collarbone causing a heavy arm afflicted with pain, numbness, and tingling. Even though thoracic outlet syndrome was first described in 1956, one of the best weapons against thoracic outlet syndrome was first recorded in 2600 BC.

And what is this weapon? Armrests—because they prevent "droopy shoulder syndrome."

Do your shoulders droop? Droopy shoulders crowd the space between the first rib and collarbone, known as the thoracic outlet. This space becomes even more crowded during pregnancy as the baby pushes upward. Neither nerves nor blood vessels like cramped quarters, and they will let you know it in the form of pain.

The simple cure for this type of irritation is armrests, but not just any armrest will do. If the armrests are too high, the neck will appear short, and the shoulders get pinched. If the armrests are too low, the collarbones slope downward or appear horizontal, and the shoulders droop further.

Armrests can come in a variety of forms. If the armrests are not adjustable, try using a pillow placed on your thighs to achieve good support. This works great in the car. While standing, place your hands in your pockets. While sleeping on your side, use a pillow placed in front of your chest for the top arm to rest on.

All forms of armrests do the same thing: They take the weight off the drooping shoulders and give the sensitive nerves and blood vessels a welcomed relief from a tight thoracic outlet. Give a lift and get relief.

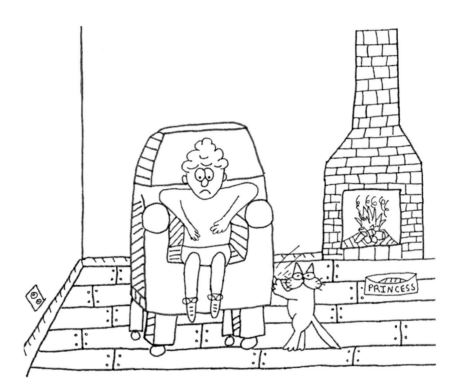

Tugging and Shrugging

Not only do these sensitive nerves become angry nerves in crowded places, they also hate gravity tugging on them all the time.

Imagine the nerves are like rubber bands coming out of the spine and down the arms. Tugging on these "rubber bands" causes a majority of the thoracic outlet symptoms. Nerves do not like sustained tension, called neurotension, because it creates nerve pain, also called neuropathic pain.

Two types of women will experience this type of burning, itchy, and/or numbing pain down the arms. One type is the young woman with a poor, lazy posture who has allowed her shoulders to droop. The second, most common type is the middle-aged woman who is losing the battle with gravity. Both types of women would benefit from the second weapon in the arsenal against thoracic outlet syndrome—shrugging.

Technically, shrugging is elevating the shoulder blades with the strong trapezius (neck) muscle. The shrugged shoulder protects the nerves from tension and pressure. Maintain a slightly shrugged shoulder (collarbones should always appear to gently slope upward) and fully shrug before any heavy lifting. Both strategies require good trapezius muscle function and can eliminate the mysterious thoracic outlet syndrome that has tormented women for centuries.

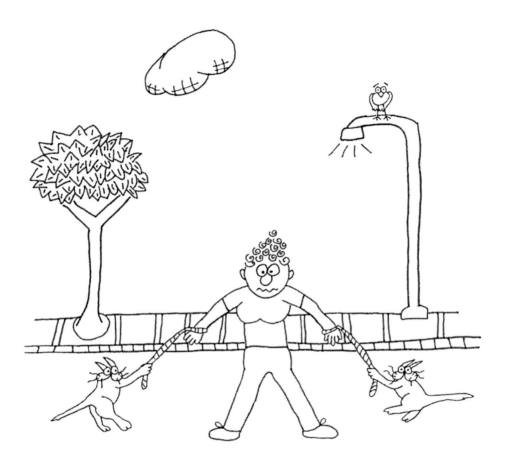

OSTEOPOROSIS

Prevention Starts in Childhood

Osteoporosis is thought to be a condition that affects older women because they lose up to half of their bone mass after menopause. In reality, women need to think about this condition much earlier—while we are raising our children.

Our peak bone density is reached by the age of thirty-five. The more bone you start with, the less impact the declining bone mass will have on you in your later years. It is like having more money in the bank—a very good thing.

The deposits start in childhood. Poor calcium intake in children leads to low peak bone densities and eventually osteoporosis. The recommended calcium intake in children (4–8 years) is 800 milligrams per day (mg/d). The recommended calcium intake for adolescents (9–18 years) is 1300 mg/d. Wow! That is a lot of chocolate milk.

Mothers are the agents for changing their children's diet and need to be part of the fight against osteoporosis. Let's talk about the grocery cart again. Buy juices fortified with calcium, snack cheese, and good old-fashioned milk. If you make calcium accessible, the kids will eat it.

Mothers can also be great role models as the kids follow their lead in eating calcium-rich foods. The calcium needs of women vary depending on the situation. Keep 1200 mg/d in mind for yourself, as that number will not lead you astray. A milligram of calcium now for you and your child is worth a pound of medicine in the future.

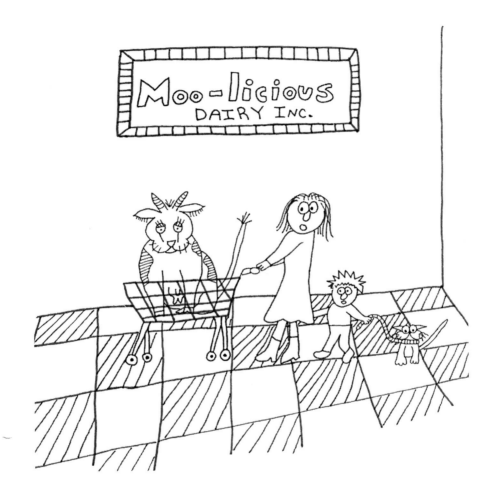

Bone Health before Medicine

Pharmaceutical companies would like to sell you a pound of medicine judging by all the commercials selling Fosamax, Boniva, and others meant to treat osteoporosis. Before accepting the risks of medication, you should think about optimizing health first.

As we now know, bone health begins in childhood. In adulthood, what should you do if you have just received the diagnosis of osteoporosis? Exercise (yes, our favorite word!) is the answer because high-intensity, low-repetition exercise can be as good or better than medicine at improving bone mass.

Bones respond to the forces of exercise by forming new bone. Specific exercises that put more arch and less abdominal crunch into your back are preferred to minimize the risk of fracture and to improve posture (see exercise Two at the end of this section). Exercise can also improve leg strength, thereby minimizing your fall risk. Falls are the single biggest hazard when your bones are weak and fragile.

Interestingly, vitamin D supplements may also reduce your fall risk by improving muscle performance. Vitamin D is a great idea for improving bone health because it works with calcium. In fact, calcium supplements are worthless without vitamin D. Even though most of our natural vitamin D comes from the skin being exposed to sunlight, today's world of skin protection requires more vitamin D diet supplementation.

Good nutrition and exercise are really better than anything the pharmaceutical companies are pushing. Before you take that prescription to the pharmacy, ask yourself, "How else can I improve my bone health?" Improving health naturally should always come before medicine.

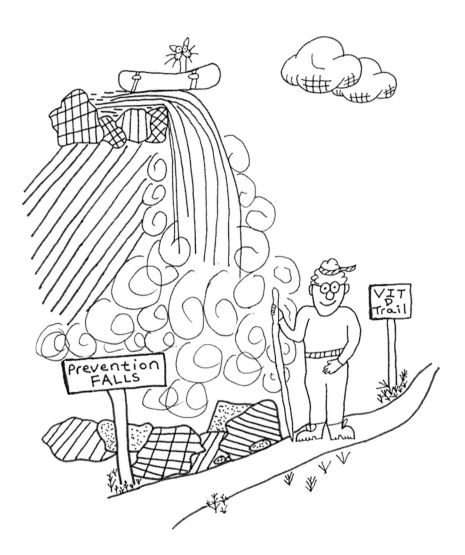

CONCLUSION WITH TWO FOR YOU

Many rewards can be found by focusing your attention on the middle child of the spine, the thoracic spine. When focusing on the gender-biased issues of osteoporosis and thoracic outlet syndrome, you can use bone health and strategic weapons such as armrests and shrugging to overcome these diseases.

To focus on preventing a stiff hump, women can outsmart mysterious thoracic spine pain with reminders not to slouch and with tennis balls (an exercise against the wall). Our own mothers may not have been given the right pearls of knowledge, but we can apply these useful hints to our children and ourselves. When put to good use, centuries of knowledge can be worth more than a whole cabinet full of medicine.

Now that you have the key information, you may be able to reduce or prevent thoracic spine pain. Give yourself a gift with these exercises for the thoracic spine.

One

This exercise stimulates some key muscles to lift the weight of the world off your sensitive nerves in the thoracic outlet. A small effort can produce wonderful results with diligence and repetition.

Two

I call this the "superwoman" exercise because it makes the thoracic spine feel super and strong. This can also open the thoracic spine to more mobility. Fly free like a bird. (If having both arms straight in front of you hurts your shoulders, try placing your hands on top of your head while lifting your elbows toward the ceiling.)

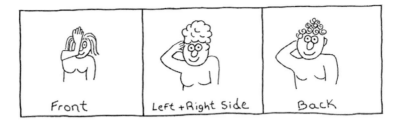

| Front | Left + Right Side | Back |

① Place hand on front, side or back
 of your head

② Push head and hand against
 each other, keeping neck still

③ Repeat each 10 sec hold
 5 times on each side

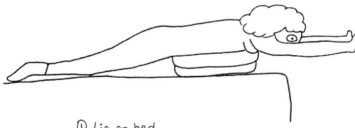

TWO

① Lie on bed
② Stack 2-3 Pillows under your
 Chest
③ Hold Arms straight out
 in front of you with thumbs up
④ Hold thirty seconds

Lumbar Spine Pain

INTRODUCTION

"Out of the blue" is where many people think lumbar spine pain (see the Navigation Page) comes from, including Lynn.

Lynn is a healthy twenty-nine-year-old with no worries about her aging spine. Despite the occasional twinge in her low back over the past five years, she has continued to bend at the waist frequently, sit for hours on end, and reach for everything without moving her feet.

Although spinal disc degeneration is usually without symptoms in the third decade of life, it is not without warning signs of impending danger.

One day Lynn picked a piece of paper up off the floor and "Wham!" The back attack hit her "out of the blue." Actually, she failed to recognize the warning signs from her body, and an accumulation of "straws" is what finally broke her back. The bending, sitting, and reaching finally tipped her over the edge toward pain.

Are you on the tipping point? Are you teetering toward a back attack? Even if you are not, all women need advice about living with an aging spine and keeping themselves on the pain-free side of life.

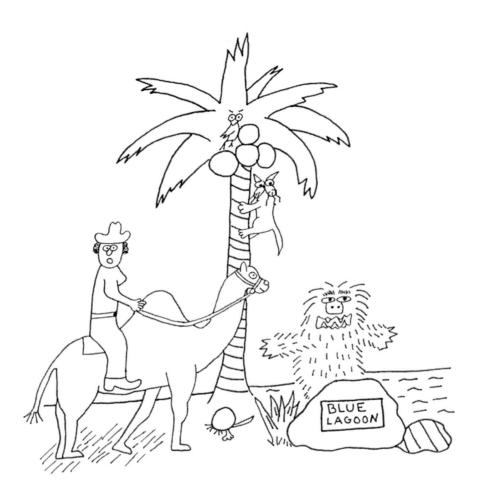

THE BUTT

Base of Support

The strongest muscle in a woman is the uterus, and the laziest is the butt or, more specifically, gluteus maximus, gluteus medius, and gluteus minimus. All three of these muscles make up what we call "the butt," and one of their biggest jobs is to help support your back.

The gluteal muscles also operate the hip in three different directions: backward, to the side, and rotationally. If the butt muscles become lazy, the whole system falls apart starting with the hip and low back. In short, if you sit on these muscles all day, they relax, stretch out, and forget their jobs. The "ladylike" (crossed-leg) position is even worse because the butt muscles get stretched further. Before you know it, the sedentary butt becomes weak and unable to support the back.

Even an otherwise fit athlete at a collegiate level is not immune to a weak butt because an injury to a knee or ankle can start a process of developing weakness in the butt as she favors one side. In fact, a woman athlete with low back pain is very likely to have developed weakness in her butt beforehand.

The butt muscles are the central link in the chain of events in which injury leads to weakness and then to low back pain. So go ahead, give those gluteal muscles a squeeze. Wake up your butt while you read; otherwise, you may develop a weak link.

A lack of butt activity may also be inherent in the fact that we are programmed to conserve energy. For example, we bend over at the waist to pick things up off the floor instead of squatting, which is healthier. Energy efficiency is good for the environment, but it is bad for your low back.

Proper back protection requires the use of the powerful, high-energy butt and legs to squat. Proper back protection requires you to override the lazy tendencies of the butt because bending over at the waist loads the hinge point of the lumbar spine right above your tailbone (see Navigation Page). The hinge will eventually wear out if the butt muscles do not get to work.

Go ahead and give them a reminder squeeze frequently for a few seconds throughout the day.

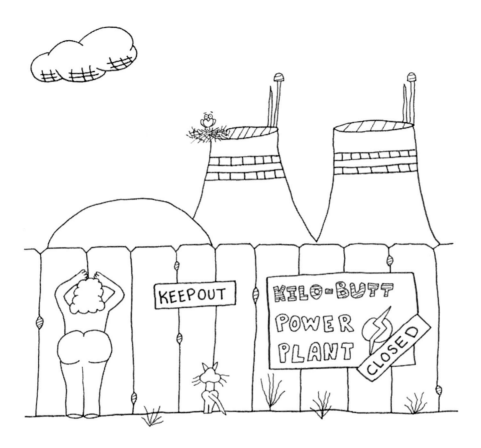

Single Leg Balance

Did you ever try to see how long you could stand on one leg in grade school? This schoolyard stunt assesses the strength of your butt.

In the doctor's office, we call this the Trendelenburg test. You fail the test if you cannot stand on one leg or if you cannot hold your pelvis still. Failure means that the butt muscles are weak.

Most people do not understand the importance of standing on one leg, but if you think about walking, you are either standing on one leg or the other. If you cannot stand on one leg with some level of stability, then you waddle. Oh yes, you will recognize the butt waddle when you see it. Work it, girl!

That sexy model waddle can really strain the lumbar spine because it twists and bends to the rhythm of the walk. The butt muscles usually prevent the low back from twisting and bending unless it is weak or the gal is making an effort to achieve the ultimate wag of her "tail feathers."

Seriously, you should continue to practice standing on one leg. In front of a mirror, try to stand for thirty seconds at a time without letting your pelvis or hips shift. Because women should not waddle like ducks, this schoolyard exercise gains adult importance as the low back ages.

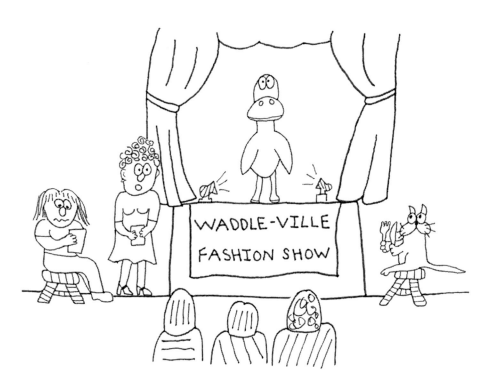

CURVES

The Hourglass

Ooo la la! Guys like to look upon an hourglass-shaped body, but some women may not like the feel of all those curves.

For many women, the chest and hips are wider than the waist and knees. This body style creates problems if you sleep on your side. When a woman sleeps on her side, the lumbar spine usually has to bend to the side in order to fill the gap left by the small waist. A whole night bending to the side makes for a stiff and painful low back. Sound familiar?

Try placing a small pillow or towel at the indentation of your waist. By filling the gap, the natural alignment of the lumbar spine is preserved.

Another curve occurs as a result of slender knees with wide hips. When you sleep on your side, the butt muscles get stretched as the top leg reaches inward to rest on the bed or on the bottom leg. An overly stretched muscle is another cause for a weak butt. Thus, women should especially consider using a pillow between the legs to compensate for the discrepancy between wide hips and narrow knees.

Body pillows also work great if you do not mind a crowded bed. The hourglass-shaped body can have its advantages; however, when it comes to the lumbar spine, curves can lead to troublesome pain unless pillows are used strategically. Properly supported alignment can tip you toward the pain-free side of life.

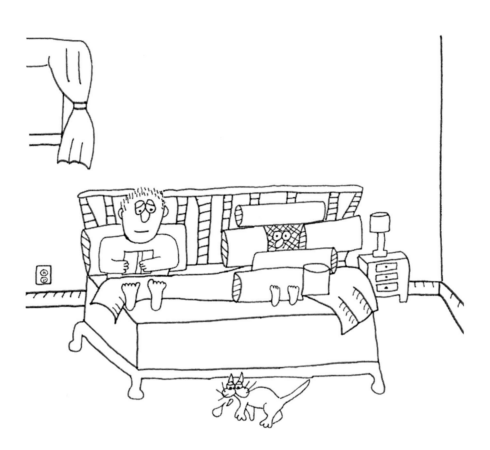

High Heels

High-heeled shoes mess with our curves and should be left in the bedroom.

Much speculation has occurred among spine specialists as to why high heels cause low back pain. Some have argued that the spiked heels offer no shock absorption, and others say that they offer no stability.

Both theories are true enough; however, low back pain occurs primarily because of the shifted body position. High heels give you a feeling of falling forward because the body's center of gravity (the plumb line) is shifted forward. Your body naturally adjusts by shifting the shoulders backward and rotating the pelvis. Otherwise you would end up on your face.

What happens to the lumbar spine in this process? Its graceful arch is lost as it flattens. Curves and arches have a mechanical purpose: to evenly distribute load. If you mess with the curve of the low back, the uneven loading leads to pain, usually because the lumbar discs are overloaded.

Teetering on the cutest shoes may not be worth an aching back at the end of the day. Vanity always has its price.

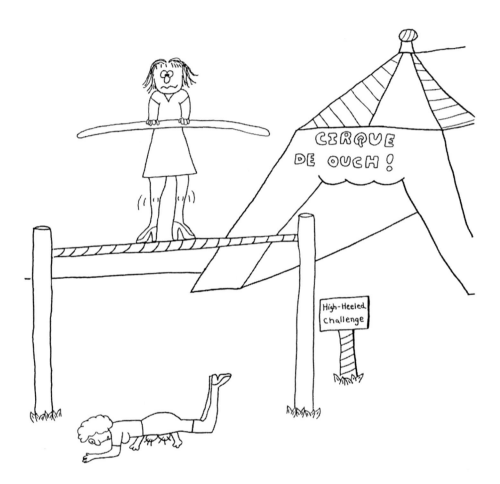

THE BABY MACHINE

Hormones

A woman's body is built to have babies. We have learned how breasts and curves can influence the spine. Let's learn about the single biggest influence on the lumbar spine—our hormones.

Unique to women, these hormones, estrogen and relaxin, allow us to have children. Estrogen not only produces our feminine features but is also a part of the menstruation cycle. Relaxin causes the ligaments to relax in the event a nine-pound baby needs to come through the birth canal.

Many women have back pain during menstruation and pregnancy because of relaxin's ability to loosen the ligaments around joints. This lack of joint stability predisposes us to injury and pain.

The estrogen factor is a bit more complicated. Estrogen products, like oral contraception and hormone replacement therapy, take the female message to the receptors, our body's mailboxes. The message found in the estrogen "mailbox" is not always friendly. For example, the estrogen receptors found on the spine's joint cartilage seem to have a toxic, degenerative effect on that joint. In fact, estrogen replacement leads to increased rates of osteoarthritis, the common breakdown of joints.

Thus, women using oral contraception or hormone replacement therapy are at higher risk for low back pain. Those women who have never used estrogen products have a lower rate of low back pain.

My advice for this complicated topic is simple: If you have low back pain, stop using oral contraception, and, later in life, if you have low back pain, seriously reconsider the use of hormone replacement therapy. Hormone replacement therapy should only be used for a short period of time, not for the chronic prevention of fracture and osteoporosis (see Osteoporosis section).

Your body has a delicate balance of hormones; add fuel to the fire and you might end up with lumbar pain.

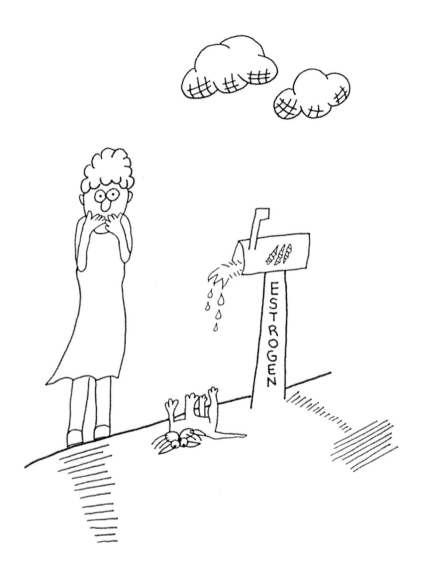

Tummies

Sometimes our baby-machine body gets stretched out of shape. Those nasty stretch marks attest to the severe change in the tummy's shape during pregnancy.

The skin is not the only part stretched beyond belief. Muscles lie just under the surface of the abdominal skin. Just as the butt muscles lend support to the lumbar spine, the abdominal muscles give a corsetlike stability to the low back. As our built-in corset, these muscles are absolutely crucial for maintaining a pain-free lumbar spine.

A previous stretch incident like pregnancy can deactivate the tummy muscles, and this inhibition leads to low back pain. The larger your abdomen during pregnancy, the more likely you are to have low back pain.

Therefore, after pregnancy, the most important exercises retrain the multiple layers of abdominal muscle that were stretched out of shape. The situation is worse if you had a cesarean section. You can just imagine the damage done when these muscles were cut.

It is never too late to get back into shape after pregnancy. Just find the time and find a program that will work for you (see suggested reading list). Pregnancy is usually the first time women experience low back pain. Turn your tummy "corset" back on, and it will be your last.

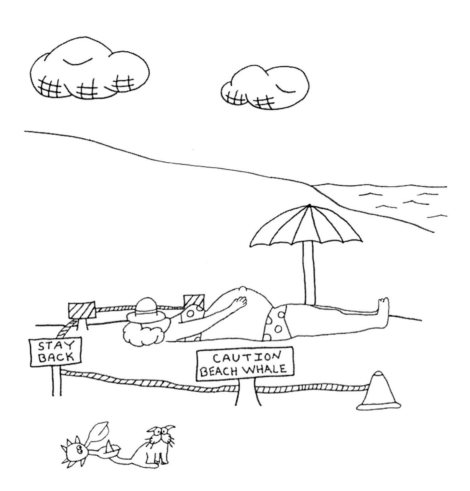

Conclusion with Two for You

Lumbar pain in women does not come out of the blue. Sometimes muscles stop working to support and stabilize the low back. Sometimes our choices about wearing high heels and using hormones adversely affect the spine.

We have no choice about the shape of our body or the fact that pregnancy happens, but we can heed the warning signs before the back attack pounces.

So the next time you are teetering on those spiked heels, remember that you may also be on a tipping point toward the misery of low back pain. It may be time to reexamine your choices, turn on the lazy muscles, and give the lumbar spine some support.

Give yourself a gift to stay on the pain-free side of life.

One

This great exercise is simple and will wake up the butt and tummy muscles. In the push-up position, imagine a glass of water is on your back. Do not spill a drop by sagging or moving.

Two

Another exercise that uses the butt and tummy muscles is called the "bridging" exercise. Give that lazy butt a squeeze to hold a solid bridge.

ONE   TWO

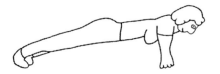

1) Assume push-up position
   resting on fists
2) Squeeze Butt,
   Hold 30 sec
3) Do not let back sag
4) Repeat

*Added Challenge: Feet together

1) Lie on your back
   with knees bent
2) Lift Butt off floor
3) Squeeze Butt,
   Hold 30 sec
4) Repeat

*Added Challenge: Feet together

Triple D's for Spine Care

INTRODUCTION

Wake up, sleeping beauty; you have another opportunity for a momentous day.

As you pass by the mirror, you see a reflection of a transformed you. The exercise and good nutrition are really starting to pay off. You are slimmer, your skin looks healthier, and, most of all, you are pain free.

Every morning you have scheduled "you" time, and today your body wants a good stretch and a walk. After some fruit and yogurt, you head out the door with your shoulders back, your head held high, and a smile on your face. Your pace is steady as you carefully try not to hurry or waddle. The new shoes feel great with plenty of cushioning.

Mentally, you clear your mind of worries about the past or the future. A deep breath allows you to live in the moment with no fear because life is much better now that you have learned the three *D*'s for spine care—depressurize, desensitize, and develop.

Mirror, mirror, on the wall, now I am happy once and for all.

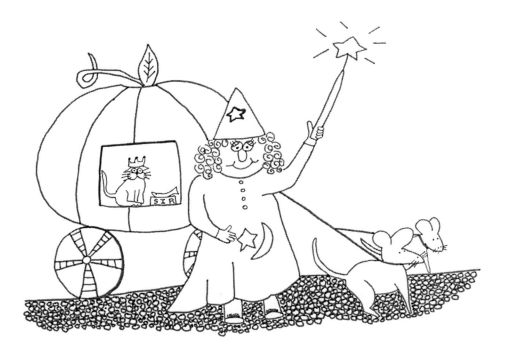

DEPRESSURIZE

The Spine

The spine lives under pressure, especially at the base of the neck and at the base of the low back. These high-pressured areas are the first to wear out, which is why we have talked extensively about creating a good base of support in the shoulders or the butt.

This wearing-out process starts with disc degeneration. As the disc degenerates, it dries out like a piece of wood. Just like wood, a dried-out disc develops tiny fissures. Put that poor little dried-out disc under pressure, and you are asking for trouble.

The discs are in between the spine bones like little balloons that can literally pop under pressure. Not only does pressure cause physical stress, pressure also causes chemical stress in the form of inflammation. Inflammation is your body's chemical reaction leading to pain, swelling, and redness.

Controlling the pressure is essential for treating spine pain by reducing inflammation. How can you depressurize your spine? Many people rely on tractioning with systems that stretch the spine by hanging or pulling, but before you get too fancy or expensive, understand that pressure builds up throughout the day based on your activities: Lying down has the lowest pressure on the spine, sitting a moderate amount, and bending forward a high amount.

Spending all day in higher pressure positions such as sitting or stooping leads to increasing pain toward the end of the day. Unless you manage the pressure throughout the day, your spine will pop.

To manage building pressure, you may need to lie down or traction periodically. Even a relaxed walk can relieve pressure when done in moderation. However you choose to do it, you need to depressurize the spine.

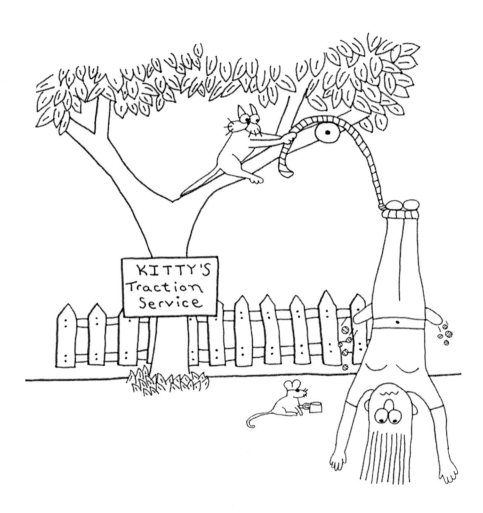

Pressure Chamber of Life

Not only do you need to depressurize your spine, you need to depressurize yourself.

We have talked about our tendencies as women to "do it all" and worry about everyone but ourselves. All of this emotional pressure translates into highly tense muscles.

Where do you feel the tension? Your neck? Your low back? Yes, your spine will take the brunt of your stressed-out life. Tension builds up in the large, powerful spine muscles, which act like vise grips on the bones, ligaments, and discs. Remember, these tissues can only tolerate so much pushing, pulling, and squeezing before they become painful.

The moment you start to feel bad physically and/or emotionally is the moment you start to slouch and carry yourself like a turtle because posture reflects attitude. Shy or negative attitudes cause unhealthy spine postures and eventually pain.

Because life is a pressure chamber, you must take the time to decompress or you will pop. Hobbies or other pastimes you enjoy are a great place to start decompressing. Hugging someone you love is a great way to depressurize at the end of the day.

Depressurize is the first *D* for treating spine pain.

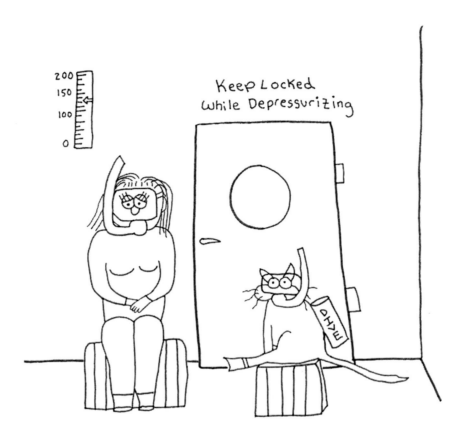

DESENSITIZE

The Nervous System

Nothing likes to be confined or stretched for indefinite periods of time, especially the nerves.

Previously, you read about how brassiere selection and use of armrests can help the nerves feel better and less irritated. Expanding on this concept of nerve sensitivity leads us to a process called sensitization.

Nerves have a certain threshold at which point a stimulus will create a painful signal. As a nerve becomes irritated, the signal threshold lowers to the point that normally nonpainful stimuli such as light touch or stretch will cause pain.

An example of sensitization that most people have experienced is a sunburn. Sunburned skin does not like to be touched for quite a few days until the nerves have a chance to calm down.

We can evaluate the amount of sensitivity in the nervous system by intentionally stretching a nerve. If the nerve causes pain with slight stretch or movement, then that nerve has been sensitized. A sensitized nerve creates painful signals during normal activities such as walking, sitting, or reaching.

Nerves that become irritated with normal movement need to be desensitized. Desensitization is used in psychology to cure phobias, and you can desensitize your nervous system in a similar manner by gradually reintroducing movement.

Desensitization can begin with walks as short as one minute or even by visualizing yourself on a short walk. Over the following weeks, slowly increasing the time spent moving will help you to desensitize your nervous system.

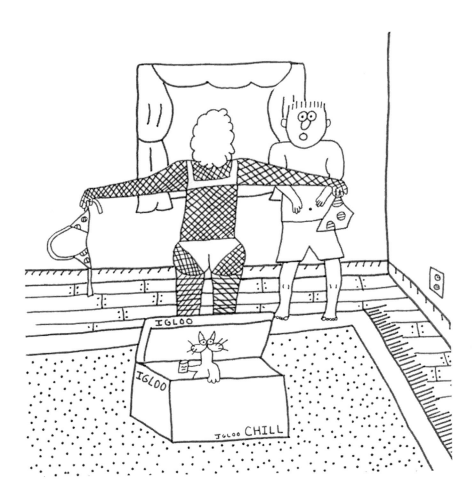

You

Some people are more sensitive to pain than others, and women certainly get tagged with the "sensitive" label. The reality is that women are not simply overemotional; women actually respond to pain differently.

Some women avoid moving because it causes pain. These are the women who do not necessarily feel more pain, but they respond by avoiding it. This behavior is called the fear-avoidance behavior.

As a general rule, most women are not confrontational and like to avoid conflict. This inherent nature causes us to be labeled as being "more sensitive" to pain because we respond to it with avoidance rather than confrontation.

Whether or not you choose to respond to pain with confrontation or avoidance depends on how much you fear pain. Remember the vicious circle of pain and fear. Fear of pain hinges on the meaning or significance we assign to the pain. If all headaches mean that you have a tumor, then the resulting fear will cause you to avoid anything that might trigger a headache. A pain that does not seem life threatening is more likely viewed as a nuisance that does not interfere with normal activity.

Desensitizing from pain is really just disconnecting from its imagined meaning of importance. You do not need to be psychic to know that not all headaches are tumors. Someone who lost her leg and has "phantom" leg pain can tell you that not all pain is from actual tissue damage.

In reality, some pain needs to be confronted or ignored. By creating a new reality about pain, you can desensitize yourself.

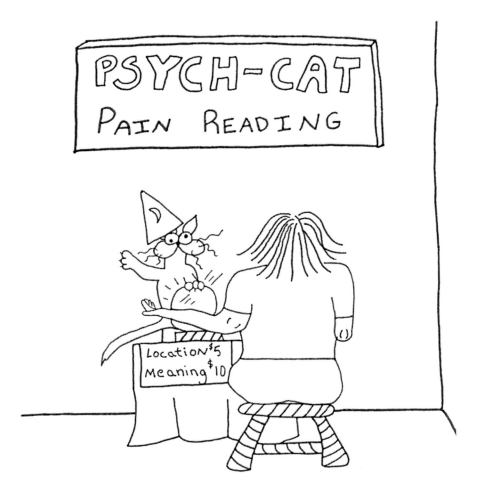

DEVELOP

Good Support

The spine needs various types of support from armrests to butts. All techniques I have mentioned in previous sections are physical supports.

High heels and poorly fitting bras offer the wrong type of support. Pillows, well-adjusted headrests, and strong muscles offer the right type of support. Even with good physical support, dealing with a spine problem can be very isolating and overwhelming.

Although millions of people experience spine pain, you may feel like the sole victim in that boat. Your physician may be too hurried or lack understanding. Your spouse may not know what to do. Your family may just need you to get better.

Sometimes what your spine needs is a little emotional support. Most women have good social networks, but spine pain can force you to avoid going out. This isolation leads to depression. Depression and pain create yet another vicious circle in which one makes the other worse.

Please do not get trapped in this cycle; use your support system or develop a better one. Invite friends over or find an activity that you can do, whatever it takes to put a smile on your face. A daily dose of smiling can be just what the doctor ordered.

Developing a good physical and emotional support system for your spine will help you when you eventually do have to row your own boat.

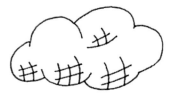
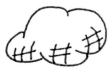
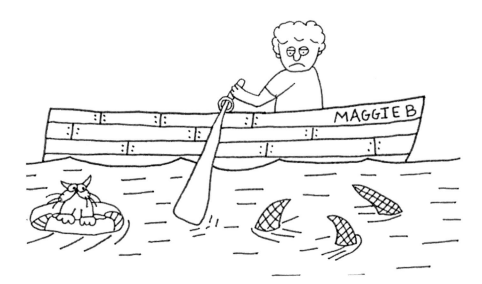

Good Habits

Amazingly, many people do not equate bad habits like smoking, eating snack food, and being physically inactive with pain. Good habits such as exercising to learn a body language and getting enough calcium for strong bones begin in childhood. Mothers are the best role models for good habits, but sometimes mothers do not have the best habits themselves.

Now is the time to reevaluate your habits for the sake of your children and yourself. What type of physical or mental habits do you have that can be improved for better health?

Pain can be a doorway to transform all of these habits. If you are lucky enough not to have pain, then this can be an opportunity to prevent it. Of all the habits that I have mentioned, mental habits are the ones that can really be a roadblock to recovery. Worry and negative thoughts can become a mental landslide in the multitasking, caretaking woman who has to "do it all."

Do you fit the anxious woman profile? You will stay connected to the pain if you allow anxiety, depression, and fear to amplify it. With the right mental habits, a negative thought can be replaced by a positive one. With some deep, deliberate breathing, you can learn to live in the moment instead of worrying about the future or the past.

You may be the pillar of good physical health, but poor mental habits can undo all of that. Take the time to develop well-balanced, good habits that can clear your path to a happy spine.

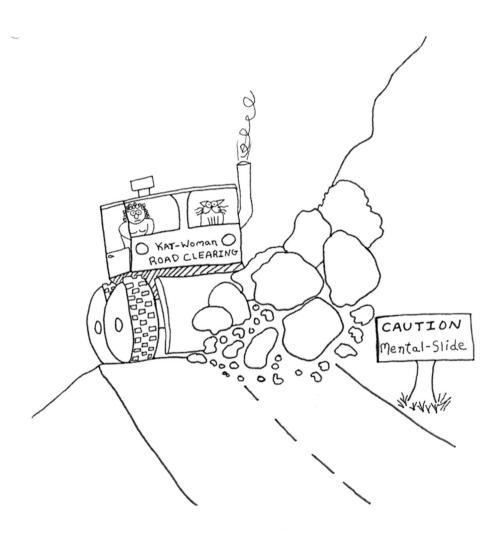

CONCLUSION WITH TWO FOR YOU

Depressurize, desensitize, and develop are the three *D*s of spine care because our sensitive system will break under the pressure of poor support and bad habits.

Magic wands do not exist, but the three *D*s can help your wish for a healthier spine come true. Good advice can be magical, especially when tailored to you as an individual and as a woman.

Health care can no longer treat men and women equally because the gender differences greatly impact the treatment of spine pain. Women should not be underestimated. Women should not accept gender-generic advice. Women need gender-specific advice from high heels to hormones about their spine.

Give yourself these final gifts and pass the pearls from this book to another woman who needs woman-to-woman advice about her spine.

One

The weakest butt muscles demand more attention. The simplicity of this exercise is astonishing. Just bend your knees so that the bottoms of your shoes face the ceiling. The sides of your shoes should be touching. Gently, press your feet together. Bingo, the butt muscles turn on. The results can be dramatic when combined with all of the previous exercises into a daily routine.

Two

Tapping into the basic instincts can be extremely powerful in rehabilitation. An exercise on breathing and balance round out your "you" program. Make sure to schedule a "you" session daily.

ONE

TWO

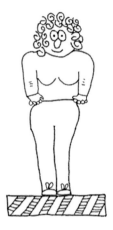

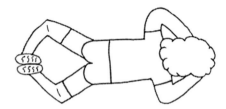

1) Lie on your tummy
   with knees bent

2) Spread legs apart

3) Push feet together for 30sec

4) Repeat

1) Stand on Cushion with
   feet together

2) Take a Deep Breathe
   thru your nose

3) Exhale thru your mouth

4) Repeat

*added bonus: try with eyes closed

Suggested Reading

Explain Pain by David Butler, 2003, Noigroup Publications, Australia.

Spinal Stabilization: The New Science of Back Pain by Rick Jemmett, 2001, etc. Press Ltd., Canada.

Bounce Back into Shape After Baby: From One Mom to Another by Caroline Creaser, 2001, Executive Physical Therapy, Inc., Colorado.

Sex and Back Pain: Advice on Restoring Comfortable Sex Lost to Back Pain by Lauren Andrew Hebert, 1952, 3rd edition 1992, Impacc USA, Maine.

7 Steps to a Pain-Free Life: How to Rapidly Relieve Back and Neck Pain Using the McKenzie Method by Robin McKenzie, 2001, Plume (Penguin Group), New York.
All are available at www.OPTP.com.

More suggested reading and useful websites can be found on my clinic website, www.gvbacks.com.

Notes (arranged by appearance)

General Health for Your Spine

Benson, Dave. "The Title IX law changed the perception of female athletes." *The News-Sentinel,* www.FortWayne.com.

U.S. Department of Labor. Title IX, education amendments of 1972; Section 1681.Sex.

Cassell, Eric J., ed. *The Nature of Suffering and the Goals of Medicine.* New York: Oxford Press, 2004.

Ornish, Dean. *Love & Survival: The Scientific Basis for the Healing Power of Intimacy.* New York: Harper Collins, 1998.

Scott, S.C., M.S. Goldberg, N.E. Mayo, S.R. Stock, and B. Poitras. "The Association Between Cigarette Smoking and Back Pain in Adults." *Spine* 24 (1999): 1090–1098.

Akmal, M., A. Kesani, B. Anand, A. Singh, M. Wiseman, and A. Goodship. "Effect of Nicotine on Spinal Disc Cells: A Cellular Mechanism for Disc Degeneration." *Spine* 29 (2004): 568–575.

Kjaer, P., T. Bendix, J. Sorensen, L. Korsholm, and C. Leboeuf-Yd. "Are MRI Defined Fat Infiltrations in the Multifidus Muscles Associated with Low Back Pain?" *BMC Medicine* 5:2 (2007): 1741–7015.

Weil, Andrew. *Healthy Aging: A Lifelong Guide to Your Physical and Spiritual Well-Being.* New York: Alfred A. Knopf, 2005.

Yaffe, K., A. Kanaya et al. "The Metabolic Syndrome, Inflammation and Risk of Cognitive Decline." *JAMA* 292 (2004): 2237–2242.

Cervical Spine Pain

Stemper, B., N. Yoganandan, and F. Pintar. "Gender and Region Dependent Local Facet Joint Kinematics in Rear Impact." *Spine* 29 (2004): 1764–1771.

Yoganandan, N., S.A. Knowles, D. J. Maiman et al. "Anatomic Study of the Morphology of Human Cervical Facet Joint." *Spine* 28 (2003): 2317–2323.

IIHS News Release, www.hwysafety.org/news_release/2004/pr111404.htm.

Leinonen, V., M. Kankaanpaa, M. Luukkonen, M. Kansanen et al. "Lumbar Paraspinal Muscle Function, Perception of Lumbar Position, and Postural Control in Disc Herniation-Related Back Pain." *Spine* 28 (2003): 842–848.

Wilson, S. and K. Granata. "Reposition Sense of Lumbar Curvature with Flexed and Asymmetric Lifting Postures." *Spine* 28 (2003): 513–518.

Lee, J., D. Zava, and V. Hopkins. *What Your Doctor May NOT Tell You About: Breast Cancer.* New York: Grand Central Publishing, 2005.

Survey at www.Maidenform.com.

Harbo, S., E. Jorum, and H. Roald. "Reduction Mammaplasty: A Prospective Study of Symptom Relief and Alterations of Skin Sensibility." *Plastic and Reconstructive Surgery*, January 2003.

Chadbourne, E., S. Zhang, M. Gordon et al. "Clinical Outcomes in Reduction Mammaplasty: A Systematic Review and Meta-analysis of Published Studies." *Mayo Clinic Proceedings* 76 (2001): 503-510.

Thoracic Spine Pain

Sahrmann, S. *Diagnosis and Treatment of Movement Impairment Syndromes.* St. Louis: Mosby, 2002.

Sapsford, R., J. Bullock-Saxton, and S. Markwell. *Women's Health.* Philadelphia: WB Saunders, 1998.

Cleland, J., J. Childs, J. Fritz, J. Whitman, and S. Eberhart. "Development of a Clinical Prediction Rule for Guiding Treatment of a Subgroup of Patients with Neck Pain: Use of Thoracic Spine Manipulation, Exercise, and Patient Education." *Physical Therapy* (January 2007).

Meneck, J.Y., M. Requejo, Kulig. "Thoracic Spine Dysfunction in Upper Extremity Complex Regional Pain Syndrome Type I." *Journal of Orthopedic & Sports Physical Therapy* 30(7)(2000): 401–409.

Lindgren, K. "Conservative Treatment of Thoracic Outlet Syndrome: A 2-year Follow-up." *Archives of Physical Medicine and Rehabilitation* 78 (1997): 373–378.

Lindgren, K., E. Leino, and H. Manninen. "Cervical Rotation Lateral Flexion Test in Brachialgia." *Archives of Physical Medicine and Rehabilitation* 73 (1992): 735–737.

Brantigan, C., and D. Roos. "Diagnosing Thoracic Outlet Syndrome." *Hand Clinics* 20 (2004): 27–36.

Pynt, J., J. Higgs, and M. Mackey. "Milestones in the Evolution of Lumbar Spinal Postural Health in Seating." *Spine* 27 (2002): 2180–2188.

Ide, J., M. Yamaga, T. Kitamura, and K. Takagi. "Compression and Stretching of the Brachial Plexus in Thoracic Outlet Syndrome: Correlation Between Neuroradiographic Findings and Symptoms and Signs Produced by Provocation Manoeuvres." *Journal of Hand Surgery* 28B (2003): 218–223.

Cyriax, J. *Textbook of Orthopedic Medicine*. London: Bailliere Tindall, 1947, 9th edition 1998.

Crosby, C., and M. Wehbe. "Conservative Treatment for Thoracic Outlet Syndrome." *Hand Clinics* 20 (2004): 43–49.

Rizer, M. "Osteoporosis." *Primary Care Clinics in Office Practice* 33 (2006): 943–951.

Winzenhberg, T., E. Hansen, and G. Jones. "How Do Women Change Osteoporosis-Preventive Behaviours in their Children?" *European Journal of Clinical Nutrition* (2007): 1-7.

Heaney, R. "Bone Health." *The American Journal of Clinical Nutrition* 85 (supp) (2007): 300S–303S.

Lumbar Spine Pain

Nadler, S. "Relationship Between Hip Muscle Imbalance and Occurrence of Low Back Pain in Collegiate Athletes." *American Journal of Physical Medicine and Rehabilitation* 80 (2001): 572–577.

Millisdotter, M., B. Stromqvist, and B. Jonsson. "Proximal Neuromuscular Impairment in Lumbar Disc Herniation." *Spine* 28 (2003): 1281–1289.

Lateur, B., R. Giaconi, K. Questad et al. "Footwear and Posture." *American Journal of Physical Medicine and Rehabilitation* 70 (1991): 247–254.

Opila-Correia, K.A. "Kinematics of High-Heeled Gait." *Archives of Physical Medicine and Rehabilitation* 71 (1990): 305–309.

Franklin, M., T. Chenier, L. Brauninger et al. "Effect of Positive Heel Inclination on Posture." *Journal of Orthopedic Sports Physical Therapy* 21 (1995): 94–99.

Ha, K., C. Chang, K. Kim et al. "Expression of Estrogen Receptor of the Facet Joints in Degenerative Spondylolithesis." *Spine* 30 (2005): 562–566.

Felson, D. and M. Nevitt. "The Effects of Estrogen on Osteoarthritis." *Current Opinion in Rheumatology* 10 (1998): 269–272.

Rosner, I., V. Goldberg, and R. Moskowitz. "Estrogens and Osteoarthritis." *Clinical Orthopedic and Related Research* 213 (1986): 77–83.

Brynhildsen, J., E. Bjors, C. Skarsgard, and M. Hammar. "Is Hormone Replacement Therapy a Risk Factor for Low Back Pain Among Postmenopausal Women?" *Spine* 23 (1998): 809–813.

Musgrave, D., M. Vogt, M. Nevitt, and J. Cauley. "Back Problems Among Postmenopausal Women Taking Estrogen Replacement Therapy." *Spine* 26 (2001): 1606–1612.

Wijnhoven, H., H. Vet, H. Smit, and S. Picavet. "Hormonal and Reproductive Factors Are Associated with Chronic Low Back Pain and Chronic Upper Extremity Pain in Women—The MORGEN Study." *Spine* 31 (2006): 1496–1502.

Dull, P. "Hormone Replacement Therapy." *Primary Care: Clinics in Office Practice* 33 (2006): 953–963.

Hodges, P. and C. Richardson. "Inefficient Muscular Stabilization of the Lumbar Spine Associated with Low Back Pain." *Spine* 21 (1996): 2640–2650.

Ostagaard, H.C., G. Andersson et al. "Influence of Some Biomechanical Factors on Low Back Pain in Pregnancy." *Spine* 18 (1993): 61–65.

Triple *D*'s for Spine Care

Wognum, S., J. Huyghe, and F. Baaijens. "Influence of Osmotic Pressure Changes on the Opening of Existing Cracks in 2 Intervertebral Disc Models." *Spine* 31 (2006): 1783–1788.

Miyamoto, H., M. Doita et al. "Effects of Cyclic Mechanic Stress on the Production of Inflammatory Agents by Nucleus Pulposus and Anulus Fibrosus Derived Cells In Vitro." *Spine* 31 (2006): 4-9.

Wilke, H., P. Neef et al. "New In Vivo Measurements of Pressures in the Intervertebral Disc in Daily Life." *Spine* 24 (1999): 755-762.

Butler, David. *The Sensitive Nervous System*. Unly, Australia: Noigroup Publications, 2000.

Butler, David, and Lorimer Moseley. *Explain Pain*. Adelaide, Australia: Noigroup Publications, 2003.

Fritz, J., S. George, and A. Delitto. "The Role of Fear-Avoidance Beliefs in Acute Low Back Pain: Relationships with Current and Future Disability and Work Status." *Pain* 94 (2001): 7–15.

About the Author

Christina Lasich, MD, is a concerned physician with spine pain herself who has a valuable message for all women ready for a healthier spine. As an award-winning graduate from the University of California, Davis, School of Medicine, Dr. Lasich draws her expertise from years of experience as a solo practitioner in the field of spine rehabilitation. She loyally resides in her hometown with her husband on Brown Dog Ranch.

Lumbar spine pain has been a part of her life for nearly twenty years. Although the pain provided roadblocks in her career, first as a firefighter, then as a physician, she has transformed into a happier, healthier person. From one woman to another, in this book she would like to pass some pearls of wisdom to you. For more information about Dr. Lasich, please visit her Web site, www.christinalasich.com.

978-0-595-46891-1
0-595-46891-8

Printed in the United States
109366LV00001B/1-80/P

9 780595 468911